I0766824

DON'T BE *a* PRETTY FAT GIRL

How to Go from a Size 16 to a Size 6 in 6 Months

NEYSA LEICHER

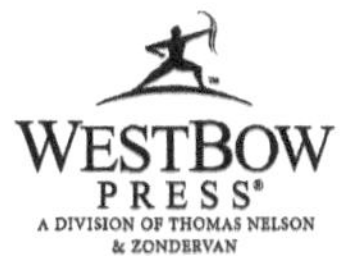

WESTBOW
PRESS®
A DIVISION OF THOMAS NELSON
& ZONDERVAN

WestBow Press books may be ordered through booksellers or by contacting:

WestBow Press
A Division of Thomas Nelson & Zondervan
1663 Liberty Drive
Bloomington, IN 47403
www.westbowpress.com
1 (866) 928-1240

ISBN: 978-1-9736-3376-1 (sc)
ISBN: 978-1-9736-3377-8 (e)

Library of Congress Control Number: 2018908162

Print information available on the last page.

WestBow Press rev. date: 11/12/2018

DEDICATION

This book is dedicated to all you wonderful ladies who are struggling with weight loss. I hope that you will find the motivation and determination that you need in this book to reach your weightloss goals.

I want each of you to stop hiding behind you baggy sweat pants, your basketful of excuses. You can lose the weight that hinders your self esteem.

I suffered for years with weight gain until the on day that I finally realized that the key to my weight loss was right in my hands. I had never wanted it bad enough before. I was not willing to make change my new best friend.

I wish each of you the very best in your weight loss journey and hope that you will find a new love for life, your self and your family. Yes it is a challenge, but anything worth having has a cost.

Good luck to each of you I wish you the best. Enjoy your new life ahead!

PREFACE

This book is for all you ladies young and old who struggle with weight loss. I am 57 and all my life I have struggled with my weight. But finally, I figured out the answer to losing the weight and keeping it off. I will talk to you in this book exactly the way I have talked to myself. Therefore, please do not wear your feelings on your shoulder, or you will find yourself offended and never lose the weight you need to lose. So please put on your big girl panties and hold on as I guide you through the steps that helped me finally be able to lose weight. Always check with your doctor to ensure you do not have a medical condition that is your weight gain culprit. You must be careful because like myself we all look for some excuse as to why we are overweight. The truth is, most of us are overweight because we are to lazy and un-disciplined to take the necessary steps and life changes to get that extra weight off. I am excited to lead you thru this wonderful and exciting journey of weight loss. You will be glad you traveled this journey with me.

CHAPTER 1
"The Decision"

Before you can accomplish anything in life you must make the decision. Your family can't make the decision for you. Your doctor can't make the decision for you. Your spouse can't make the decision for you. Only you can make the decision.

STEP 1

This step can be a hurtful moment in your life, but it is the First step. If you don't take this step, you are already defeated. You must decide just like I did that you hate the way you look. It must be a strong hate. You must feel disgusted with yourself when you look in the mirror. When you reach this point, you are on the way to losing all those extra pounds. Like I said I am 57. I have aged fairly well. I have always worked at looking nice and taking care of myself, except for my weight gain. Who wants to be a "Pretty Fat Girl" We have all heard people make comments about someone, " she is so over weight, but she has such a pretty face" Well who wants to just have a pretty face? We can't all look like fashion models, but we can look our best.

You must stand in front of a full-length mirror nude and take a long look at yourself. Take a look from the front angle, side angle and back angle. What do you see? What does your spouse or significant other see when they look at you? No matter how much your spouse loves you, every man or woman wants to be proud of the way their spouse looks. And you deserve to know that your spouse or significant other is proud of you.

Until you feel a deep-down sickening disgust with yourself, you are not ready to lose the weight.

I have spent years being that "Pretty Fat Girl". When we took a family vacation to the beach,I would always find myself having to hide and cover up, while my family was having fun running up and down the beach,,.or playing in the pool.

I did not want to embarrass myself, my spouse or my children. Ladies whether you realize it or not your children care how you look, especially if you have boys. My 2 sons have always wanted their Mom to look pretty when we go somewhere together.

My husband and I love to cruise. A cruise is our favorite vacation. I got so tired of always having to hide myself and never being able to swim or get in the hot tub because I was "Pretty Fat Girl". No one wants to look at rolls of fat and cellulite while they are vacationing. Yes, ladies I did the same things that you do, keep a wrap on until I was ready to step into the pool or hot-tub. I would look around until no one was looking and then drop the wrap and jump into the water as fast as possible to keep anyone from seeing me. Oh yes,don't forget how we disguise the fat as we lay in the lounge chair. Your stomach sinks in and you prop your legs up to make them look slimmer. You feel so embarrassed by the way you look.

Come on ladies …. everyone knows the tricks of the trade. Stop fooling yourself… you are nothing more than a "Pretty Fat Girl".

Let's Recap Step #1

You must hate the way you look!! This must take place, or you can never move to step #2

Look in the mirror, what do you see?

Hate, disgust, embarrassment?

Great, you are now ready to get on your wonderful and exciting journey of weight loss.

THE DECISION
STEP #2

Now it really gets exciting after you have decided that you hate how you look. You must be willing to make the necessary changes to lose the weight.

You must be willing to completely change your life and turn it upside down and inside out to lose the weight. You must be tough!

If you are not willing to make all the necessary changes and sacrifices required, then stop reading this book, throw it in the trash and go get a large chocolate milkshake and continue to be a "Pretty Fat Girl".

You might be thinking that these decisions are difficult. Well, yes they are but they are necessary ig you want to lose the weight. After these first 2 steps it begins to get much easier as we continue our journey.

When I tell you, it requires changing your life, that is exactly what I mean.

You might say I have a husband, I have kids, I work every day. Look these are the exact same excuses that I made for years. You are no different from anyone else. You have 24 hours in every day.

Now – you can and should ask your family to respect your decision o make changes in your everyday life to lose the excess weight, but don't expect it. They might be all on board for a while but then the new will wear off and you must make it on your own.

Just because you have a family to prepare meals for is no excuse for you to eat the same things that you prepare for them. If you do, you will remain a "Pretty Fat Girl".

Losing the weight and becoming the best, you can requires change. The word change scares people. Do not be afraid of change. Change can be a very good thing. Change must become your best friend on your weight loss journey.

We will discuss meal planning later in this book.

How are you doing so far? Are you with me? You must accept Step 1 and Step 2 to continue your wonderful and exciting journey called weight loss.

LETS REVIEW….

1. You must hate the way you look.
2. You must be willing to turn your life upside down and inside out.

If you have truthfully accepted Step 1 and Step 2 you can now move on. If you are not fully committed at this point do not continue wasting your time by continuing with this book. You must accept Step 1 and 2 before you can go any further.

Let's go girl!! Pull up your boot straps and let's move on. Don't settle for being a "Pretty Fat Girl.

CHAPTER 2

Things to be Aware of

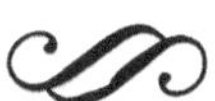

In the previous chapter I mentioned you can't expect your family to take the journey with you. You are the only person that can take this journey. Be prepared to take the journey alone with or without support from your family and friends. Yes, I hope your family supports you, but if not, go the journey alone.

Your eating habits will have to change drastically. I work in sales and investigations. I spend most of my time living in my car it seems. Some days I may do surveillance for 12 to 14 hours straight without the opportunity to eat a good balanced meal. I have found myself always in a hurry, grabbing fast-food and running to the next appointment. THAT HAD TO CHANGE!! We will discuss later ideas that can help you plan and pack your daily meals.

As a wife or mother, we feel the obligation to feed our family what they like to eat and rightly so……but remember you are on a weight loss journey, not your family.

Do not expect them to eat the way that you do.

Now comes the exciting part. You must prepare food for your family that you may not be able to eat while on your weight loss journey. What I found is that I have helped my family eat healthier simply because I was eating healthier. But again, this is your weight loss journey, not your spouse's, not your kid's. Remember as you prepare food for you family, Step 1 and Step 2. Do you want to just be a "Pretty Fat Girl?"

Weight loss is all about choices. Remember ……change is your best friend.

ME + CHANGE =BFF

We will discuss in detail later about food choices.

The thing to remember now is you must be willing to prepare your food differently from your family's food. This may require getting up a little earlier or staying up a little later. I promise you the results are worth the effort.

REMEMBER- Change is your new best friend!!!

TIPS:

Do not sample what you are preparing for your family. This can add many unwanted calories with just one small sample. Have your family sample it for you if you feel that it must be sampled. If you MUST sample it, ONLY touch it to the end of your tongue. Remember this journey is about YOU and reaching your weight loss goals!!!!

Sampling can be a terrible downfall especially if you cook a lot.

You have 2 choices:

Don't sample or

Sample and continue to be a "Pretty Fat Girl"

Every step I am giving you is a step that I had to make to start and continue my personal weight loss journey. I am not telling you to do something that I have not already dome. Believe you me, the results are worth the change.

REMEMBER…..CHANGE+ ME = BFF

Don't sample left overs. When you clean off the table and empty off the plates, DO NOT eat or sample any food left on your family's plate. I grew up being taught that we should always clean our plate and not waste any food. If kids left any food on their plate Mom always ate it to keep from throwing it away.

THROW IT AWAY!!!!!!!!

Do not eat it. Your eating the scraps does not help the staving people in the world, it only makes you a "Pretty Fat Girl".

While you are preparing your family's meals this is a great time to sip on a glass of water with lemon, unsweet tea or a diet soda. That will help you to not feel deprived while you are preparing their meals.

It is a Must that every day you weigh and look in the mirror at yourself,in the full-length mirror- nude. This allows you to see all the fat, cellulite and thing you need to work on. If you do not see the fat, it is hard to take the weight loss journey.

CHAPTER 3

GUILT

One of the most difficult things for me was guilt. I would find myself feeling guilty if I took time for myself. I would be at the track walking and start to worry about getting home to my family. Let me assure you that your family will appreciate you taking the time to make yourself look better. Remember that your family wants you to look nice. You must have guilt free time!

I would be at the gym working out then find myself cutting my workout time in half because of guilt. I felt like I needed to hurry home to cook, wash clothes, help with homework or just be there. I am not saying that you should neglect your family, you must find time for both. Many times, I would wait and go to the gym after energy level is lower, and you do not have as productive of a workout. Remember that change is your new best friend unless you want to continue to be a "Pretty Fat Girl".

Don't feel guilty, as you take care of your self and lose the weight. You will feel much better, and have more energy to care for your family.

CHAPTER 4
IT'S ALL ABOUT YOU

After Step 1 and Step 2 this might just be the most important step for you to take, especially if you are a lady reading this book.

YOU MUST FOCUS ON YOU

1. Try to be as pretty as possible at ALL times even if you are not going out anywhere.

2. Spend time reading beauty and fashion magazines. When you watch television, watch shows with fashion and beauty. You can get

inspired by keeping up with the latest trends in fashion and beauty. Do not be afraid to try something new (hair, makeup or clothing)

REMEMBER…. CHANGE IS YOUR NEW BEST FRIEND

3. Window shop. Look for those pretty outfits that do not fit your size yet. Imagine yourself in that "sexy little black dress". In a few short months you can be the one wearing it.

Go ahead and pick out that swimsuit that you have always wanted to take to the beach this summer. Keep it out so that you can see it every day. Try it on once a week. That will help to motivate you to reach your weight loss goals.

Take that beauty or fashion magazine and pick out that model you want to look like, that will help to motivate you. If you need to put her photo on your refrigerator door, bathroom mirror, dash of your car or somewhere you will see it over and over each day so, that each time you want to eat you see that photo to help keep you motivated. You are well on your way!

Try on those high heeled shoes you would love to wear, but feel your weight prohibits you from doing so.

Add color to your wardrobe. Don't be afraid to wear bright colors. The bright colors will empower you and help keep you motivated. Never let your age hinder you from trying new things! I am 57 and my daughter is 26 we share shoes, jewelry, pieces of clothing etc.

CHANGE IS YOUR NEW BEST FRIEND

THROW AWAYT YOUR SWEATPANTS!! They are your worst enemy. Throw away any other loose and baggy clothing that you have. As ladies we have hidden all our fat under loose (comfortable) clothing for long enough. Expose your fat. Do you want to be comfortable, or a pretty fat girl?

If you are not constantly reminded of your fat you will lose direction or your journey. GET RID OF THEM NOW.

Wear clothing that reminds you of your fat, so you will stay motivated to get rid of it.

Something that worked great for me was to go and pick out a beautiful sexy dress that is one size smaller that what you currently wear. It needs to be one that you just love. Something you can fee beautiful and sexy in. Take a photo of yourself, remember it should be to small right now. Imagine the day the dress will fit you. Keep that photo hanging in a place that you will see it numerous time each day, maybe in your closet or on your refrigerator. Allow yourself to look forward to the day that you can wear the dress in the near future. If it is only 1 size to small, so you will probably be able to wear it next month. If your budget is tight, shop at second hand stores. You can find many beautiful outfits at resale shops.

Do not forget to look nice under your clothing also. Go to a lingerie shop and find nice underwear. Throw away your "granny panties" find something nice and sexy that will fit your body and make you feel good about yourself. Just like with your clothing, find something that does not fit yet and keep yourself motivated to reach your goal, so you can fit into it soon. I am sure that your spouse would love to see you in a nice sexy gown instead of sweat pants and a tee shirt.

NOW, here starts the excuses. I just can't afford a new dress. Fine, it can be new to you. Shop yard sales and thrift stores. Thrift stores are full of nice clothes. Also, there a social media sights that sell clothing at a fraction of the new cost. Find something that makes you feel beautiful and sexy. I have shopped second hand stores all my life. Don not make excuses!!! People who succeed, find a way to do so. NO EXCUSES.

Do you want to just be a "Pretty Fat Girl?" This is also a great time to experiment with new makeup trends and hairstyles. Go have a facial done. If you have a teenage daughter, ask her advice on makeup changes for you. Go to the makeup store and have the sales person help you with different makeup options. This is all about change. Remember that change is your new best friend. Go bold with a new hair style or color. But make sure you always use a professional. Try a new nail color. Get a membership at the local tanning salon.

CHAPTER 5
EXERCISE

If you are not used to an exercise program always consult with your doctor before starting a program. Everyone's body responds to exercise in many different ways. You will have to find the way that your body responds to best.

For me, I love walking as my main exercise. I like to walk outdoors when possible instead of on a treadmill. Because each of us are difference I am going to tell you what my routine was. I walked each day. I started with

¼ mile then went to 2 miles each day. On days when I have extra time I would walk more than 2 miles. The more you walk the more you lose. Also walking helps to make your posture better and makes you steadier on your feet. Then I would also go to the gym each day and work with weights. I personally go every day, but you can do every other if you have to. I would do a leg workout, arm workout and full body. There are many trainers that can give you pointers on how to conduct a weight workout. I found that doing both walking and weights expedited my weight loss. Exercise + healthy eating = weight loss. There is no easy method for losing weight. It takes work and dedication.

I have a lot of people ask me about taking supplements and such for weight loss. I am not opposed to that. I actually have taken some natural products from the local health food store to boost my metabolism. Some people need that extra boost to get their metabolism revved up to burn all the extra fat. That is a decision that you and your doctor will have to make.

CHAPTER 6

FOOD AND DIET

We have all heard the saying, "you are what you eat" well I believe to a degree that is true. There are many diet programs available that limit carbs, fats, calories. What ever works for your body is fine. Personally, I do better on a low-fat diet that I do a low carb. You will have to find the meal program that works for your body metabolism. Regardless of your program you must stay away from sugar and heavy starches. Throw away the chips and cookies. Nibble on veggies. Drink your coffee black. I use artificial sweetener in my coffee and tea. Drink lots of water. I like low fat cheese and cottage cheese. Beware of fruits due to the high sugar content. My diet mainly consists of all type meats, low fat cheeses, sugar free drinks, veggies, salads, eggs, fish. There are many recipes out there for fat free or low carb eating. I always treat myself one meal a week when I go out with my family and have any meal that I want. BUT ONLY 1 meal each week. I do not eat after 7 pm. If I feel really hungry I will have a drink or treat myself to a cup of sugar free ice crème. I like to pour cold coffee over the ice crème or some grape juice to add favor. (easy on the grape juice due to sugar calories) Again everyone's body responds differently to types of foods. So, you have to find what your body responds to best. Bottom line— always cut calories. Most anyone will lose weight on a typical 1000 calorie a day diet or less.

I hope that everyone who reads this book can obtain the needed motivation and inspiration to reach their weight loss goals. I am no different than any of you. I had to find motivation to keep going each and every day. Allow yourself to be creative in what you do. Find what works for you and stick to it. When you reach your goals, you will be much healthier and happier which will allow you to be a better wife and mother. I had to over come each obstacle that you face. That is why I was so passionate about writing this book as a motivational help for each of you.

You must decide that you hate the way you look. That is the only way you will ever decide to make a change I found that my biggest problem was staying motivated Staying motivated = losing weight. Do not let others discourage you….you have to do it for yourself. You are worth the effort.

Each of us is made differently. You may lose weight differently than your friend does. Do not compare yourself with them. Accountability to a weight loss partner can help keep you motivated. It is always nice to have a friend to walk with or work out at the gym with. But if not……do it on your own.

IN REVIEW:

Decide you do not like the way you look. You must have a deep, sincere disgust with the way you look.

Make the decision to change. Realize that you CAN look nice and lose the weight.

Be willing to do whatever is necessary to reach your goals. Do not let anything stop you from reaching your goals. This is about YOU. Take this time to help yourself, in turn you will be helping others. MAKE this special time for you.

Understand that you may take the journey alone. If you have a weight loss partner, that is wonderful. If your family supports you, that is great….but if not take the journey alone. It will be the best decision you have ever made.

Keep yourself motivated. (find that person you want to look like, choose that sexy little black dress, pretty dainty underwear, change your hair and makeup) Go outside your comfort zone. Do not worry about what others think. This is your journey. It is all about you. Be bold and brave.

Remember that change is your new best friend. Life is all about changes. This is just one of the many changes you will face in your lifetime. But this is the most important change you will ever make.

Post photos on your refrigerator and places you will see throughout the day. Do not worry what others say. This is one of the most important steps to keep you motivated.

Plan that beach vacation with your new swimsuit. Plan your trip for a few months away, this will give you something to look forward to.

Tell yourself its all about you. Remind yourself that you are bold and beautiful, that you can make these changes to have the body that you want.

Most of all NEVER, NEVER, NEVER give up!!!

Keep this book on your night stand or in a place easy to find. When you feel discouraged pick it up and read through it again. I specifically designed it to be easy to read and short enough that you can use it as a motivational manual.

Decide today that you can be whatever you want to be. Pull up your boot straps, put on your big girl panties and GO GIRL. Accomplish your weight loss dreams.

You too can go from a size 16 to a size 6 in 6 months!

Don't settle for being a "Pretty Fat Girl"

FINAL THOUGHTS

I hope that you have reached your goal, whether it be 10 pounds or 100 pounds. You are worth the effort.. Each time someone tells you how nice you look, you will forget all the effort that it took to get that way. The benefits out weight the things you had to give up.

I hope that you will make this a new way of life for yourself. If you do, you will never be worry. You will be proud of yourself and so will your family and friends, You will find such a difference in your state of mind, your energy level and your overall wellbeing.

Do not allow yourself to become satisfied. Always be striving to look nice or you will slip back to the way you were," A Pretty Fat Girl".

Enjoy your new-found energy and stamina. Plan those trips you want to take. Look at yourself in the mirror and tell yourself you are somebody, you are beautiful and enjoy your new body.

It will continue to take motivation in order to maintain your weight loss. It is a lifelong challenge. Make it fun along the way. Plan your girls trip, plan the trip with your daughters. Now you can have the energy to spend fun time with your grandkids. ENJOY your new body and life.

If you ever find yourself feeling sluggish and not caring how you look any more, if you find yourself wanting to cheat on your new life style pull this book out and read it all over again. Sometimes that cheesecake plays with our mind. Just remember where you came from an where you are now. Do whatever it takes to keep yourself motivated to maintain this new body that you now have.

Remember- change is your new best friend!!!!!!

Never be afraid to consult with a doctor is you feel that your body will not lose weight. There is always a possibility there could be a health issue that causes that, Many people just need the help from a weight loss doctor to go along with their life change. This is all about YOU, make your dreams come true....... ENJOY THE BEACH